# The Terminal

**BY: SARAH BRADEN**

Founder of Our Terminal

First paperback edition July 2020

Cover and interior design by Megan Sjuts (Building 07)

ISBN 978-0-578-70131-8

Published by Our Terminal

www.ourterminal.com

# Dedication

It's with great tenderness that I release our story into the world. Your life well-lived, your love for those around you, and your courage in the face of suffering and death will be an encouragement to all who face their own terminal journey. Thank you for showing us how to live life to the fullest until the end. I love and miss you every day.

# Journeying Through Terminal Illness With Hope & Each Other

# Contents

# Foreword

If you are holding this book in your hands, you are - most likely - staring a terminal diagnosis in the face. Whether it is you who has been given the diagnosis, or a loved one sitting beside you, your thoughts, feelings, and disbelief are probably all-consuming.

I have felt those same feelings, too.

When a doctor says there is no cure,  the natural (and sometimes immediate) response is an onslaught of real, raw emotions, many of which you have likely never before felt to this magnitude. In the midst of those feelings, as long as life continues, you must face every moment of every day… physically moving step-by-step and emotionally processing the things that come your way. This will not be easy. It might be one of the hardest things you ever have to do.

When Mom got sick, I went through a long, soul-searching process of trying to make sense of it all.  I wondered why — why was this allowed to happen, why our family, why now?  I was angry, overwhelmed, and fearful about what was to come. I was exhausted, at times lonely, and often felt too weak to do what was required. Some days I was too numb to feel anything at all.

BUT, beneath it all, there was hope. Deep, consistent, never-forsaking hope. The kind I had known all my life but had never had to rely on until faced with mom's diagnosis. And with this hope, came peace. Not the kind of peace that promised everything would be okay, but the kind that reminded me God was with me in the storm. He wasn't going to leave us alone on this road. My prayer is that, no matter what you face today, no matter how hard the circumstances or how scary the emotions feel, that peace can be a companion for you and your loved ones, too.

As I share our story with you, there are two things I would like to note in advance:

First, as much as I saw God work in and through this diagnosis, it wasn't without hardship. I loved my mom dearly; but, at times, our relationship was complicated. The last several years of her life were filled with many happy memories, as well as some deep pain. Perhaps you are coming into this chapter of life with wounds from family relationships. The idea of caring *for* your loved one, or being cared for *by* your loved one might feel too vulnerable or difficult. I understand that, too. Watching a loved one die is one of the most gut-wrenching experiences we can go through. But, in my experience, it can also be one of the biggest privileges, greatest blessings, and most redemptive parts of your life.

No matter what your relationships look like, *hope* is available to us all in this final stage of life. I will talk more about that idea throughout this book.

Second, your story will look different than mine. The circumstances surrounding your life will be unique to you, and your family dynamic will be special as well. That said, as you walk yourself or your loved one to the end of life, I think we will find similar emotions, questions, fears, and yearnings. Each entry that I share was written during my mom's illness and is accompanied by a specific blessing I found on that day. I have also included some reflection questions which can help you process your own feelings and experiences. Following the questions, you will find a prayer that can be lifted up to God, whether this is your millionth prayer uttered or your very first.

Through reading this book, I hope you find that you aren't alone in this trial. One of the reasons *Our Terminal* exists is to connect you to people who have walked this path before you — people who understand the pain, the wrestling, the responsibility, and the courage it takes to keep moving forward every day. Ultimately, my biggest prayers are that you will meet and know the perfect Helper, Companion, and Savior, waiting to walk with you every step of the way. That God, the Creator and Author of your life and story, can bring you hope along the winding path that is to come. And that you will know you are loved, carried, and comforted by a loving God as you navigate this terminal diagnosis.

With love,

*Sarah*

# I Didn't Sign Up for This

At the tender age of eighteen, I traveled to Slovakia alone. Just graduating high school, I felt mature, independent, and carefree. And having traveled internationally several times before, I was excited to spend three weeks at a camp with teenagers from all across the globe. In the naivety of youth, I had no anxiety or fear. I was on top of the world and untouchable.

But two weeks into the trip, I found myself needing emergency medical attention. The Slovakian goulash contained just the right concoction of ingredients to jumpstart some previously undiagnosed food allergies. With the camp nestled on top of a rural hillside, the nearest hospital was two hours away. Fear began to creep in. The staff called a doctor who lived one village away. Quickly traveling the dirt roads to my camp, she threw me into her car and monitored my breathing on the winding road to the hospital. As we pulled in front of the dilapidated building, I shuddered to think about what level of care might be available in this run-down, Communist-era building. I was far from home... and I was scared.

Conversation took place between my rescue driver and the attending physician as I was led to a room. Naturally, I couldn't understand a word of what was spoken and after getting me undressed and settled on a cot, my driver announced she had to return to her clinic and would have to say goodbye. Staring at her in blank silence — unable to process the reality of what she said — I was engulfed by the intense realization that I was completely alone. The tears started to fall.

From where I lay, I had a clear view into the doctor's private office. Following his initial examination, he receded back behind the quiet confines of his desk, reading through medical textbooks and plucking away on a manual typewriter. I was growing increasingly anxious. Thankfully my life wasn't in imminent danger; but as he read and typed, my tongue sat swelled inside my mouth. Not knowing what was wrong with me, panic began to set in. And all I could do was wait.

After some time, the door to my room opened, and I saw that my new roommate had just arrived. As they completely undressed this large man in front of me, I realized that I had also lost my privacy. Rolling onto my side, I felt the journey couldn't get much worse. The seconds turned into minutes. The minutes turned into hours. I didn't have a phone. I didn't have a friend. All of my expectations for this international adventure melted into a puddle of tears on the bed.

Finally, the textbook and typewriter seemed to whisper a plan into the doctor's ear. Up he rose from his chair, striding across the room to a wall of cabinets and drawers. Watching in horror, the doctor pulled out a bin of needles... needles that were unwrapped, unprotected, and potentially unclean. He prepared the IV bag right in front of me and I lay on my rickety cot and sobbed. Helpless and afraid, I came to terms with the fact that I might end up with a disease born from a dirty needle. This was a life-changing moment for me. I was no longer in control and I knew it. I turned on my side as the IV punctured my skin. As I ran my finger down a foot-long crack in the tiled wall beside my head, all I wanted to do was go home. I didn't sign up for this.

After some time, my tongue deflated and my airways were opened. The medicine had worked. But the wounds lasted longer. Mental wounds over the trauma of seeing my naked roommate. Emotional wounds over the unknown risk of contracting a disease. Wounds over being abandoned in a moment of need. Wounds over my disappointment of a carefree trip gone horribly wrong. My hopes were high and the disappointment was great when life handed me a different plan.

Life is full of expectations. We dream big dreams in the quiet moments as we lay down to sleep.

*I didn't sign up for this.*

We plan, create, and strive as we look ahead to the future and only see a clear, well-traveled path with bright, happy milestones ahead. So when disaster hits and the realities of life take over, we are often left feeling cheated. What happens when life takes you someplace you don't want to go? What if your expectations go unmet and you end up confused, bewildered, angry? What if you find yourself on a road you never wanted to travel in the first place?

## QUESTIONS:

Do you remember a time when your neatly-made plans went awry? If so, how did it make you feel? How did you respond?

Have you ever looked back and found any positive aspects to unmet expectations?

When things don't go as planned and your circumstances feel shaky, where do you find your hope and assurance?

**IF YOU WOULD LIKE, LET'S PRAY THIS FIRST PRAYER TOGETHER.**

*Dear God, for some of us, prayer is a familiar part of our life and for some of us this is the very first time we have talked to you. Whether it's our thousandth prayer or our first, we acknowledge that we are on a trip we never signed up for and walking down a road we hoped to never travel. This unexpected diagnosis has entered our lives in a way that is shocking, overwhelming, and uncertain. As we walk through the pages of this journal, help us to see you at work in our own story and help us to develop a deeper hope and trust in you. Amen.*

# About My Mom

People die. This is the reality and the part of life that I struggle with most. I imagine many of you do, too. Having lost several people close to me, including one friend at just thirteen years old, I've attended many funerals, seen lifeless bodies laid to rest, and been exposed to the pain that overtakes when life is cut short. Death is what I dread most and what I can't seem to escape. Fear of dying, or losing another loved one, has held me secretly captive. It has influenced my decisions, prevented me from taking risks, kept me in bondage to fear.

Several years ago I lost my mom to a brutal and unforgiving cancer — watching her die, slowly and painfully, before my eyes. My life changed forever by escorting her to death's door and releasing her into eternal life. She showed me what it meant to live life well to the very end, modeling how to have courage in the midst of the worst-case diagnosis and the hardest days that followed. Her faith, how she trusted Jesus in the midst of her suffering, helped me to do the same. The outcome is that fear is no longer my default. Safety is no longer my top priority. Comfort is no longer my focus. My heart is at peace.

As long as I can remember, Mom was a faith-filled person. She valued God, the church, and the impact both could have on her kids. However, it wasn't something we ever discussed, not something we ever read or prayed about together; not something I had seen her fully embrace. But as cancer came knocking on her door — as her body was physically weakening — she was growing stronger daily in faith and in wisdom. She cherished the story God was writing through her terminal cancer diagnosis and yearned for Him to use her illness for good. One day she said to me, "Sarah, you need to write a book." And so, wholeheartedly believing her legacy isn't done and that people's lives can be impacted by her story, I am sharing our journey with you. Because peace can be your companion, too... no matter what you face today and what you will face in the days to come.

***

Mom was the most courageous woman I have ever known; a strong, determined fighter of two separate breast cancer trials and a final encounter with pancreatic cancer. Her humor, bravery, unpredictable spontaneity, and self-confidence didn't wane even as cancer presented every type of obstacle. Her courage bred resilience not only in me but in others who faced similar diagnoses and trials of various kinds. Mom cared, not only about her own experience with cancer, but about other people's as well. She wanted each person she came in contact with to see her smile and know that they weren't alone in their story.

When I think of Mom, my mind floods with things she valued. Here are just a few...

For one, she unashamedly invested in black Toy Poodles. Her first poodle puppy (regally named Baron Phillipe) joined the family soon after my parents got married and each poodle that followed had a royal title added to its name. Baroness Colette, Countess Monique, Lady Bridget, Duke Ferdinand, and Queen Isabella scurried in groups around our house; they were esteemed in her eyes. About a decade into this poodle "collection," my mom decided to enter the breeding business, retrofitting our laundry room into a birthing center. My sister, Emily, and I later discovered one of her main motives in this new entrepreneurship was to teach us in a roundabout way about the birds and the bees. Mom hoped to eliminate any awkward conversations that could take place in our preteen years. Was it unconventional? Absolutely. But did it work? It actually did.

Chico's profited from Mom's frequent jacket purchases and Estée Lauder was the only cosmetic company that carried the perfect shade of red lipstick. Wine on the patio with friends was a highlight of her day. You could call her the hostess with the mostest. Volunteering in the community brought her great pride and much admiration from those around her. Being the PTA president, band booster club member, school's athletic club guru, hospital receptionist, and homeroom mom gave her joy and a sense of accomplishment. When the volunteer signup sheet was passed around, Mom was always the first to sign up for anything—and I do mean anything. Much to my surprise and horror, Mom appeared as a California Raisin dancer in one elementary school assembly wearing a stuffed black trash sack and green stem hat. But the embarrassment I felt sitting on the cold cafeteria floor watching her choreographed dance did not come close to the shock my sister received in junior high when she stumbled into Mom subbing for the lunch lady one day—hair net and all.

There was one thing Mom rarely worried about... other people's opinions of her. If someone needed an advocate...she advocated. If someone needed a cheerleader... she grabbed her pom-poms. If the referee at a third-grade basketball game made a bad call... she corrected him (even to the point of getting ejected from a game once). If a random Saturday night needed some action... she threw on her best Halloween costume and created the fun. From California Raisin to french fry server, Mom was comfortable in who she was created to be—friend, personal champion, and confidant to all.

As I left the nest for college, Mom sought ways to stay connected and engaged in my life and those of my friends. Driving down to Texas A&M University to watch home football games became a highlight for my parents. By day they were surrounded by the revelry of game day activities; and by night, they moonlighted as casino dealers for Pi Beta Phi sorority events. (In hindsight... maybe they just came to keep tabs on my whereabouts.) In more recent years, Mom spent her time leading social activities within her 55+ community. She was the lead fundraiser for the neighborhood annual pajama party benefiting the Susan G. Komen foundation, helping raise over $40,000 each year she was involved. It was hard to tell Nancy "no" when she asked for something.

You could find Nancy wearing dangly earrings while working in the yard and could frequently spot her at Mexi-Go, enjoying tortilla chips and margaritas alongside people she loved. Trendy clothes, favorite places, hosting, and volunteering all helped make Mom her spontaneous, spunky, one-of-a-kind self. But the thing that set Mom apart was her investment in other people. For example...

When I was in seventh grade, Mom came to me and Emily with the news that she and Dad were going on a trip. Our regular sitter was unavailable, so Mom had found an alternative. Excitement filled her voice as she described this new caretaker... someone she knew we would enjoy. She had contacted the junior high school custodian and asked her to keep us for several days. As she told us, the often-used preteen expression of "are you nuts?!" crossed our faces. Recruiting someone she barely knew to keep her kids seemed out of character. Choosing someone whose first name we hadn't ever even considered seemed irresponsible at best. We felt like this was an invasion, a trick even. Then the revelation hit — Mom did know her. While we passed this janitor day after day, never glancing her way, Mom saw her. Valuing her contribution to our school, Mom poured out love and attention as she would have for a close friend. Our custodian was well known by Mom, enough to entrust her with her most prized possessions... us. It wasn't random.

This was Mom. This is what made Mom different. This is what made Mom special. It will forever be a huge part of her lasting legacy. Mom valued people most.

# Diagnosis

In July 2013, on a family trip to Disneyland, Mom found a lump in her breast. Remission from her first cancer trial that began in 2003 had lasted ten years, and hearing that she would face another long road was discouraging and scary. Because my parents had divorced in 2009 and Mom lived alone, she decided to make a temporary move to Oregon following her double mastectomy. This allowed me and my family to care for her during her chemotherapy. After securing an appointment with one of the most brilliant and well-respected oncologists in the region, her treatment began. In good hands — the best hands — she was pronounced cancer-free at the end of four treatment rounds. We were so grateful.

The five months in Oregon had been a trial run to see if this lifelong southerner could tolerate the rainy winters and to gauge whether this was a place she could start anew. After much contemplation and prayer, the decision was made to return home to life in Texas. She packed up her things and made the return journey. Four months went by and remission and cancer became more of an afterthought as daily life and reconnecting with relationships took center stage. So you can imagine my astonishment when I received a text one morning in July that read: *I am selling my house and moving to Oregon... permanently.*

Immediately picking up the phone to clarify, I barraged her with questions. Was this the same woman who had just decided to move back to Texas? Why the sudden change of heart? Her answer was matter-of-fact, "Sarah, I just know the move is a necessity." Why she felt so strongly, no one knew, not even her. It was just a feeling that couldn't be ignored. After spending thirty-three years in Texas, leaving her community and support system to start over in a new land was a life-altering decision. Though flummoxed, we trusted her instincts and believed God had laid this on her heart for reasons we couldn't understand. I helped plan her move including finding a house just two minutes from mine; proximity was her highest priority.

An enormous moving van filled with all her belongings rolled into town on October 30, 2014. Hope and anticipation filled the air, excitement for what lay ahead. Our three daughters dreamt of sleepovers with Nana; and visions of sitting at the kitchen table doing crafts, baking cookies together, and celebrating special events danced in her mind. Images of day trips in the minivan, chats over lunch, making new friends, and setting new routines began to take shape. The first few months were just as we imagined. We enjoyed a nice Christmas in her new home.

Then on January 29, 2015, just three months after moving to town, Mom became sick with what appeared to be a stomach bug. That weekend, she curled up on our couch with Queen Isabella nuzzled at her knee, half watching the Super Bowl in a nauseated funk. It was clear that something was wrong; we just didn't know what. Eventually, we took her to the emergency room at the nearby hospital.

The ER felt harried that day and the wait was excruciating. Despite her misery, Mom managed a smile as we huddled together in a nook of the waiting room. We watched in horror as a gunshot victim came limping into the building. Feeling like it was an appropriate time for a selfie, Mom instructed me to snap a picture. When we finally moved back to a room, tests were ordered, and medications were administered. Relief began to wash over her and she fell asleep. Slipping outside to make a phone call, I took a moment to take a few deep breaths and say a prayer... "Whatever your plan is, God, I trust you."

*Whatever your plan is, God, I trust you.*

Soon after returning to her bedside, I settled into a chair as the ER doctor cautiously opened the curtain. Anticipating the results, I held my breath. He pulled up a chair, gently placing his hand on Mom's arm. She woke up. Looking her square in the eyes, he said, "Nancy, we found something and it doesn't look good."

The word cancer had reared its head again... this time in a mean and vicious way. Mom had two tumors on her abdominal wall and a spot on her pancreas. As the news sat heavy in the room, disbelief engulfed us. In that moment of diagnosis, I mustered the courage to tell her that it would be okay. That we would get her the best of care... again. That God was in control. I said that and I believed it to my core. But I also had no idea how God could or would redeem this story.

## QUESTIONS:

Everyone's path and circumstances are unique... were there any "coincidences" or "timely" things that happened right before the sickness started? Is there anything that you can see in hindsight was happening behind the scenes?

When you received the news of an unexpected diagnosis, what were your initial thoughts and feelings? Was it disbelief, anger, sadness, fear?

Oftentimes we feel like we have to be the strong one when hard news hits. Is this something you experienced or did you feel free to show your emotions?

## PRAYER:

*Oh God, these first days are hard. Disbelief is mixed with uncertainty, doubt, and fear. We don't like this road, and we don't want to walk through it. God, you created the world and everything in it. You know the number of our days. We ask that you will give us everything we need in the days, weeks, and months ahead. We pray that you will be the strength we can't muster up ourselves. Please help us to have eyes to see you as you are... a loving God who cares deeply for us. Amen.*

# Arriving at the Terminal

Mom was admitted to the hospital within several hours of her diagnosis. She was so very sick; her entire digestive system was paralyzed by the surrounding tumors. The pathology report showed pancreatic cancer, stage four. We would be lucky to have a few months left with her. Her days were numbered. It was the worst-case scenario. I sat by Mom's side day-in and day-out those first couple weeks, arriving at the hospital mid-morning and staying until the oncologist made his night rounds. Ragged, worn, and grief-stricken, the reality of the road ahead pierced us both deeply.

During my teenage years, Mom and I stopped by the neighborhood 7-11 most days after school to split a Snickers bar and Coke Slurpee, sharing details from our day. Long ago, she and her mom would sit at their kitchen table, share a Hershey bar, and dissect their days just as we did. Some of the best conversations we ever had occurred over a Coke and the last few months of her life were no exception. And though my heart filled with sorrow, beauty surrounded those precious days. Mom's shaky hand would reach for the room service phone and she would order two Cokes from the kitchen. We'd sip soda over stories and it was in these moments by her bedside that I began to witness the miraculous. Though this woman knew death was imminent, peace covered her like a warm blanket. Mom began to teach me how to die knowing Christ.

*I don't want to die, Sarah. This isn't the plan that I had. This isn't what I want.*

In all my experiences with death, I had yet to see it through the lens of someone who was dealing with a terminal disease. Bitterness, anger, questioning, and doubt were natural and expected feelings. Some people have asked if Mom ever had moments of questioning. Sure she did. Did sadness or grief ever show on her face? Occasionally. She was human, after all. In fact, the day before she took a final turn and was admitted to the hospital for the very last time, we sat across from each other on her living room sofa. Looking at me with yearning in her eyes she said, "I don't want to die, Sarah. This isn't the plan that I had. This isn't what I want." She had all the natural feelings and yet — underneath it — she was strong, courageous, and unafraid. She trusted God even when His plan for her future was so different from her own.

Mom's strength, trust, and courage helped deepen my faith in God in a new and more genuine way. Growing up in Texas, we attended church weekly along with most of our friends, yet Mom and I never had spiritual conversations. She made a decision to follow Christ when she was a teenager and spent her adolescent years involved in youth activities and church choir. But as an adult, she once told me, her faith was put on the backburner. It was present but not as active or alive as it once had been. This all changed once she knew her time on earth was short. Conversations about difficult topics flowed out of her in the most natural way. While out for drives in the country with visiting family and friends, she would shock them by bringing up desired details for her memorial service. While her companions became uncomfortable, worried she would be upset talking about the finality of her life, she herself felt anything but uncomfortable. Heaven was where she was headed and fear no longer ruled. During these final months of her life, Mom lived out her faith in a deeper, more powerful way than in all her seventy-one years combined. Through her unshakable trust, God began to redeem death. To take the sting away. To give us hope for what is to come.

Watching Mom face suffering with strength, find joy in the midst of the unknown, and love other people through her own pain made that time sacred. Dread filled my heart as I anticipated the end. The void would be immense. The sorrow deafening. And apart from her physical absence, I would also miss seeing God work in such tangible ways. Miracles, small and large, had become commonplace. The way God intervened for us was stuff I had only read about, but never believed I could experience myself. My life pre-diagnosis was fairly jam-packed as it was. But in "the new normal," the responsibilities on my shoulders were just too great. More people needed me than I had bandwidth to juggle. There were more logistics to handle than I was capable of managing. The emotions alone were a full-time job. It was the first time in my life when I truly experienced what it meant to be beyond myself. Reaching this point of desperation, a deeper dependence on God began to form. My eyes opened to how God works behind the scenes. Sometimes help came through people. Their words were comforting, their hugs genuine, and their presence ever welcome. Sometimes God's hand came through answers to prayers, big and small. God's intervention was all over the pages of this unfolding narrative.

Following chemo, Mom would usually end up back in the hospital for a few days as her body coped with the side effects. A well-worn cycle formed: receive chemo - be admitted to the oncology floor - get amazing care and medical intervention - get discharged to life at home - start to feel better - get chemo - start all over again. Mom cherished her time at home and her "good days," she fought hard to have strength to live life the way she desired. The more treatment progressed, the weaker she became; and the doctor ultimately chose to space out treatments to allow for reprieve. Sensing that she was growing weary, heart-to-heart conversations began to take shape. Did she want to continue treatment? Was she tired of this cycle of sickness? What did she want her future plan to be?

**QUESTIONS:**

What stage of the journey are you in right now?

Has anything happened that you couldn't explain or you felt was a "miracle" or "divine intervention"?

What emotions have you and/or your loved one been feeling? Are any of these surprising to you?

**PRAYER:**

*Dear God, because our story is different than anyone else's, it is hard to know what is waiting around the corner. While the emotions may not be as raw as they were initially, we still struggle some days to see any good in this terminal illness. We are tired and the day-to-day responsibilities are taking a toll. Please help us to feel the emotions as they come, allow us to process all that we are feeling, and help us to see your intervention and care for us each day. We want to trust you. Would you help us? In Jesus' name, Amen.*

# Preparing for Departure

On Monday, July 6, 2015, Mom steadied herself at her kitchen counter, whipping up dips for a dinner party at my house later that evening. As I mentioned about my "hostess with the mostest" mom, she loved a party and she was determined to personally help make this one special. Though weak and shaky throughout the evening, she stayed late to enjoy the fellowship. Eventually she asked to be taken home. The next day we were busy running errands and getting things checked off her usual to-do list. Later that evening we gathered around beautifully set outdoor tables, soaking in the night air while celebrating at a baby shower. When it was time to leave, two friends had to help get Mom into the car. Trembling and stumbling to keep her balance, her legs could barely hold her up. Thinking she had just pushed too hard and needed a very good sleep, I drove her home to sit beside her for what turned out to be our last intimate conversation.

After tucking Mom in for the night, I went home, flopped into bed, and wondered what the next day would hold. Maybe a good night's rest would refresh her and ease her unsteadiness. The next morning, after trying to call several times and not receiving an answer, I hopped in my car to check in. When I arrived at the house, I knew something was wrong. Her curtains were still drawn, Queen Isabella wasn't barking at the window, and the lights were all off. I found Mom still asleep in bed after 14 hours. Rousing her, she startled and cautiously put her feet to the floor. It was 11:45 a.m. and she was going to be late for a scheduled doctor's appointment. In the short ten-minute ride to the clinic, Mom became lethargic and barely responsive. Struggling to get her into a wheelchair, I raced into the office where the staff took charge and began preparing a bed back on the oncology floor of the attached hospital. Over the next couple of days, test results showed that the cancer was fully taking over, forming bleeding ulcers in her intestines. Mom's fight would soon be over. The doctor suggested that the family be called, forcing me to speak the words aloud… "Mom is about to die," I said over and over on one call after the next.

Mom was placed on hospice and we set up a bedside vigil. My dad and sister arrived to say their final goodbyes, staying day and night by her side, soaking in all the time they had left. Though starting to turn inward, Mom found subtle ways to let us know she was still there. She said "good morning" to her nurse, "I love you" to me, and even gave us one hearty chuckle. Being told that the sense of hearing is usually the last to go, we played music, read Psalms, prayed beside her, and reminisced about her life. Laughter, tears, prayers, and song filled the room and surrounded each of us in those final days. Every time someone left the room goodbyes were said, afraid that upon returning from lunch or a bathroom break, Mom would be gone. After over a week, while mom was still clinging to life, both Dad and Emily needed to return to jobs in Ft. Worth and Washington DC, respectively. Standing back, watching Emily say goodbye to Mom for the very last time was one of the most gut-wrenching moments of this journey.

On Monday, July 20, 2015, Mom's breathing became irregular and the oncologist said she would likely die by the end of the night. Twelve hours had passed since I had arrived at the hospital that morning. Weary and heartbroken, I couldn't stand the thought of being alone when that time came. Calling my husband, Michael, to come sit with me in those final hours steadied my anxiety and grief. Because every minute felt like an eternity and my body felt physically heavy with grief, I needed a moment to stretch my legs and I walked down the hall. As I passed the vending machine, my eyes fell upon a king-sized Snickers bar. Reruns of those long-ago, after-school Slurpee dates came to the forefront of my mind. Because of all the time spent in the hospital over the past months, I had come to keep coins in my pocket for times such as these. The coins rattled down into the machine, I bought the Snickers bar and hurried back to Mom's room. Methodically and intentionally, I unwrapped the treat as sadness surrounded me. I wasn't hungry in the least, but this was the only thing that made sense in this moment for me. "We" were eating a candy bar together, just like we always had. It was a sacred moment for me.

*She had been instantaneously healed. She was whole. She was perfected.*

At 9:55 p.m. Mom opened her eyes and looked straight into mine. Michael and I leaned in close, praying over her while we stroked her hair. We held her hands tight, told her that she was loved, said that it was okay to let go, and she took her last breath. In the twinkle of an eye, Mom saw Jesus face-to-face.

Those first moments after she died were surreal. The nurse came and encouraged us to take as much time as we needed to say goodbye. As her body lay there, a supernatural feeling permeated the room. I knew her spirit was no longer there. She had been healed. She was whole. While I knew Mom was in Heaven, on my shoulders rested a heavy weight of grief. I would never see her face on Earth again.

# The First Year

The process of grieving is slow. It has not "come and gone" as I thought it might. Places and people trigger memories. Walking into the grocery store and seeing the scones she liked to buy brings me to tears. Watching the white-haired lady fix her coffee at my favorite café makes my heart ache. Pulling out an old blanket of hers wafts her scent to my nose. I long to taste her food, especially her homemade spaghetti and flat New Mexico-style enchiladas. I would give anything to see her smile, hear her laugh, or share a chat with her. When exciting news comes, she is the first person I want to tell. When sad news hits, I long for her comforting words. As holidays continue to come and go, we are weighted with sadness for memories gone by. We're stifled by the newness of not having her with us. I miss her more than I had ever imagined, still picking up the phone to call her from time to time. Some days, her death still doesn't even seem real. In those moments I have to remind myself I'm not crazy. This is a process. This is grief.

Through all my mourning, God is showing me the beauty that can come in this time of sorrow. He is teaching me how to be still in His presence and find calm in the midst of the storm. Though Mom's death has brought the deepest pain of my life, I wouldn't trade walking with her through those last five months for anything. It was a privilege, an honor, and a gift. The caregiving and emotional weight stripped

*The hardest pain has equaled the greatest blessing.*

me of my self-reliance, and solely through God's mercy and grace and gentleness towards me, I am emerging resilient, complete, and whole. Had Mom not moved to Oregon, I would have missed everything—seeing the intimate ways God provided, the miracles He performed, and the everlasting peace He brought. And the irreplaceable time with Mom... I would have missed the most. What a tragedy that would have been. The hardest pain has equaled the greatest blessing.

The week Mom was diagnosed, a mentor gave me the task of keeping a journal. I struggled with the idea initially, because I was not accustomed to writing down my thoughts. Despite my hesitation, she encouraged me to start recording ways I saw God intervene in my day, even as simply as listing them as bullet points. Some entries were small, such as thanking God for creating sugar (sugar did lead to Snickers and Slurpees, after all!) Other entries were bigger, like my thankfulness for Mom's favorite nurse being on rotation when she passed away. This journal has helped me reflect back over the long and weary days and see that God was working amidst the pain. He was present, active, intervening, and answering prayers in ways I would have missed if they hadn't been recorded. This journal was a life-source for me, and will continue to bring encouragement as I walk this path of grief still to come.

And now my journal is open to you. Included in the rest of this book, you will find journal entries that God laid on my heart over the entirety of Mom's illness and death. In between each entry, you will find a thankful bullet point taken straight out of my documented days. As you flip through these pages, entering into our story, I pray that peace and rest will surround you.

Whether you are navigating a hard diagnosis of your own or if you are walking beside someone you love, my hope is that you will be encouraged and uplifted. And, most of all, that you will see God as the rebuilder of broken lives and shattered dreams. May you experience the Author of your life, the ultimate Healer, the Perfecter of all things. Because just as He has done for me and for my mom, He longs to do for you, too.

*See, I am doing a new thing!*
*Now it springs up; do you not perceive it?*
*I am making a way in the wilderness*
*and streams in the wasteland.*
**ISAIAH 43:19**

# The Journal

# Redefining Terminal

*Today I am grateful for the friendship of another family at our church walking through a similar diagnosis, it's comforting knowing someone else completely understands how I feel.*

**FEBRUARY 12, 2015**

Last week the oncologist delivered the news that Mom's cancer is terminal. Beginning to process what this means has left me heartbroken and afraid. This is new territory, propelling me into a long, heart-searching week of deep contemplation and prayer. As hospital time seems to slow and blur into indiscernible fragments of doctor's rounds and beeping machines, it takes a lot of effort to keep my mind focused and clear. While lying down to sleep last night, processing the day, God brought a vivid image into my mind. Clear and focused, penetrating to the core of my being, this vision felt as real to me as the pillow underneath my head.

A woman was patiently sitting on a wooden bench inside an old, weathered bus terminal. Looking around at her surroundings, she was content to wait for her next ride to appear. Sunlight poured through the windows of the station casting a brilliant glow around her head. Beauty, peace, and joy radiated around her. Traveling light with no bags in tow, she straightened her Hawaiian-print walking cane, and touched up her shiny lips with deep red lipstick.

As time passed, people came to sit beside her. Some talked about her past, asking about experiences and stories she had already lived. Others inquired about her future, where she was headed, and if she was ready for her next destination. Most of her company just sat, comfortable in simply being in the present with her, cherishing their time and good conversation. No one was in a hurry. No one seemed anxious about their impending departure. Everyone was filled with deep love and affection. Through this beautiful picture God began to reshape my idea of "terminal."

*Without fear or regret, she is neither eager to leave her past nor dreading the future, content to sit in her terminal until her departure time arrives.*

Mom is at the terminal of life—her journey on this earth isn't over. She is at a transition point from healthy years past to her eternal home waiting in the unforeseeable future. Without fear or regret, she is neither eager to leave her past nor dreading the future, content to sit in her terminal until her departure time arrives. I should not fear this terminal.

Many people don't get to ever sit in this transition point with their loved ones, never getting the opportunity to "gather 'round" one last time. To listen. To laugh. To learn. So many loved ones never get to wait patiently on the wooden bench, enjoying this sweet sliver of time together. This terminal is a gift to me, to everyone who knows and loves Mom. Hard, yes. Tears shed, many. Do I wish I could take her off the bench and firmly place her back to her past life, definitely. But I will choose to see this terminal as a gift; space where we can share memories of the past, show love in the present, and hold hands as we wait for the bus headed to her eternal home. Today the word terminal — as it helps define our terminal journey — has become one of the greatest blessings God has ever given me.

### QUESTIONS:

I am sure you felt so many emotions as you first heard the word "terminal." Reflect on some of the initial feelings you experienced here. Have your feelings evolved or changed at all in the time since the initial diagnosis? How so?

Who are some people that you would like the opportunity to "gather 'round" in this season of your life?

**PRAYER:**

*Dear Jesus, we come before you and admit that this terminal diagnosis is hard and sometimes feels impossible. If we could write a plan for our own life, this isn't what we would have chosen. It is hard to trust you when the news is harsh and the trial before us seems insurmountable. But we choose now to trust that your plan is perfect. We come near to you, God, and ask that you would reveal to us your presence intimately. Please show us glimpses of your beauty and fill us with your peace even in the midst of this trial so we will know you are near. We trust you, Lord, even when we cannot see your full plan and we may not ever see it this side of heaven. Amen.*

# Love DOES Things

*Today I am grateful for the high schooler who I mentor. Usually I am the one sending her texts of encouragement, but today she bathed me in prayer and Scripture. It was just what I needed.*

**FEBRUARY 14, 2015**

Traditions are a core part of family identity. They bind us together as they create lasting memories. Having unique ways to celebrate holidays and special ways to mark events brings unity and a sense of camaraderie. As we've grown up as a family, we have come to value these special traditions and look forward to living them out together year after year.

Valentine's Day usually consists of the girls waking up to a colorfully decorated table, filled with muffins, eggs, sausage, and juice. Handwritten cards lay on each of their plates with a small gift attached. Michael and I always pick out a Bible verse for them that will adorn their walls for the next year; we pray this reflective truth over them, as we tuck them into bed at night. We have a certain rhythm to the day. Everyone knows what will happen. We anticipate its familiar pace.

This Valentine's Day there is no decorated breakfast table. The kids did not wake up to a yummy breakfast. There were no small gifts or cards waiting for them. Their mom wasn't present either. I cried walking down the hospital wing thinking about the loss of our rhythm. I didn't even get to hug my girls this morning and I felt like I had failed them. I worried they would look back on this holiday and feel unloved or forgotten amidst the current chaos. But as I grabbed my early morning coffee and climbed the familiar stairwell to Mom's hospital room, God began to speak truth into my heart.

This year my love is more real... and it is deeper, perhaps, than ever before.

Today I am not celebrating my girls the way I want to. I am not home to kiss my husband or make breakfast. Feeling like I let them down, I ponder the idea of what love really looks like. Today I am doing meaningful and active love. Brushing Mom's hair, reading her messages, encouraging her spirit, and advocating for her care means much more than a loss of pretty plates, cards, and gifts. Though feeling like I cheated my girls out of a beloved family day, in reality, I am modeling true love to them in a different way than I ever could before.

In the Bible Jesus says, "Love the Lord your God with all your heart and with all your soul and with all your mind" immediately followed by, "Love your neighbor as yourself." And Jesus tells us to not just be hearers of His words, but doers[01]. And so we are sometimes called to give up what is known and easy and even good to love God and our neighbor. To trade out the Hallmark holiday version of Valentine's Day for actively loving my mom and showing that example to my girls. I am modeling a love that DOES things. My torn conscience has been replaced by a deep peace, and I am grateful.

*...I am modeling true love to them in a different way than I ever could before.*

My prayer is that when my girls look back on this Valentine's Day, they will remember it as the year they saw first-hand what it means to truly love deeply and sacrifice much; and that they will be spurred on to do more active love, too.

We are called to lay down our lives for one another[02], and are commanded to love one another as we would want to be loved ourselves[03]. Love God first and people next[04].

## QUESTIONS:

Who is someone that needs your active love right now? What is one thing you can do for them today that shows them you care?

_____

_____

_____

Are you experiencing any guilt or frustration over not getting to participate in or family traditions or daily rhythms? If so, what truth can you replace with those guilty feelings? *(For Example: I felt guilty and frustrated that I couldn't give my girls their normal Valentine's Day, but I recognize that the truth is that I'm showing them active love and that this season is not forever and I am doing the best that I can right now.)*

What are some expectations/hopes/plans that you might need to let go of in order to free yourself from guilt or pressure and to allow you to be present in these moments?

**PRAYER:**

*God, in the middle of all this, sometimes we just want a normal day. We want to have an easy schedule, love people in the way we are accustomed to, and feel like ourselves. In this season, those days are rare. Please help us to surrender our days to you. Help us to live with an open mind and open hands, allowing the day to come and go exactly as you plan. Help us to find ways to love those around us whatever the circumstances may be. Amen.*

# Tossed by the Sea

*Today I am grateful that I can confidently put on mascara for the first time in two weeks without fear of it immediately running off through my tears!*

**MARCH 15, 2015**

Our neighbor blessed us with a weekend away at their vacation home, located on the beautiful Oregon coastline. After discharging Mom from another grueling hospital stay, we loaded into the car and wound our way through beautiful scenery, along jagged outcroppings, adjacent to rocky seas. To say we needed this time away is an immense understatement. Watching Mom sit in front of the floor-to-ceiling windows, sewing her great nephew a baby quilt as she gazed at the open sea, is a memory imprinted on my mind forever.

As I stared out at the ocean waves today, my eyes followed a piece of driftwood. The waves would bring the wood to the surface, tossing it back and forth, slapping it mercilessly against the boulders. The driftwood had no control, no order to the churning; it was at the mercy of the next approaching wave. Right now our life as a family feels much like that driftwood. The waves come at increasingly intense intervals, sometimes ebbing for a day or two, while other times knocking the wind out of us for weeks at a time. We don't have control over the course we are charting and we often feel helpless and afraid.

Looking past the riptide and the mounting sea foam, way beyond what the human eye can realistically see, the ocean appears to be at rest. There is perfect calm in its depths. It looks quiet. It is orderly. It is still. The deep ocean water is not shaken with each passing wave.

Because I know Jesus, my life on the surface might be rocky, dangerous, and unpredictable; but beneath the raw emotions and the unyielding twists of circumstances, there is peace. I am calm. I am still. I know there is a plan in place. I hold unwavering to the hope we have been given—that on the other side of the chaos of this world we will find rest. We have been neither abandoned nor forsaken by our Creator, and the tumultuous waves will not separate us from His great love[05]. God is an anchor for our soul.

I know our family will have days of unsteady churning. We will doubt. We will cry... a lot. We will feel tossed here and there. But through it all, I will be reminded of the One who holds the ocean in His hands[06].

## QUESTIONS:

What feels like it is the most out-of-control for you right now? Is it the unexpected complications, the overwhelming responsibilities of care-giving, the uncertainty about an eternal destiny, or something else? Jot down your ideas here.

What promises of God could anchor you right now? If you don't know God personally, here are a few promises to ponder: God will never leave you[07] God has a good plan for your future[08] God sees your pain[09].

## PRAYER:

*Almighty God, Creator of the heavens and the earth, we feel tossed here and there in the emotions and circumstances of today. Steady our feet as we live out this journey set before us and help us to feel you anchor our feelings, emotions, and thoughts. Give us time to slip away and be at rest, even for just a few minutes or a couple of hours. When we get those moments, Lord, help us to remember that they are gifts from you and to spend them wisely. Please remind us today of your unfailing love in the midst of the raging, tumultuous sea of life as we now know it.*
*Amen.*

*"I am calm. I am still.*
*I know there is a plan in place.*
*I hold unwavering to the hope we*
*have been given—that on the other*
*side of the chaos of this world we*
*will find rest.*

# Life to the Full

*Today I am grateful for the handyman that asked to pray over Mom while working on her house. God is drawing people to her in remarkable ways.*

**APRIL 11, 2015**

Tonight, sitting on the lanai, watching the breathtaking Maui sunset fill the sky, I am in awe that we made it to Hawaii at all. Without the unyielding, faithful prayers of many, this dream would have only been just that... a dream. Within days of her diagnosis, Mom had made a deal with her doctor—she would supply every ounce of fight she had to get to Hawaii if he would use every tool at his disposal to support her goal. With confidence, he answered "yes." Planning this trip gave us a focus, something joyful on which to fixate our efforts. Picking out the perfect condo, planning menu choices, and selecting extracurricular activities brought upbeat conversation. For forty years, Mom had wanted to visit this tropical paradise, scheming to take the entire family "sometime in the near future." Beaches were a happy place for her, summers spent in South Padre Island, Texas were still fresh in her memory.

As the trip date approached, uncertainty reigned over if this was even possible. Mom would have a bad week, land in the hospital, and the dream trip would begin to unravel. Then, surprise! Mom would make it home and rally again. Encouragement came steadily from the doctor, saying, "Patients live longer and do better when a good goal is set before them." Calling this her "Make-a-Wish" trip, Mom bought a few new outfits and planned for perfection, despite the uncertainty of going.

The week finally came. Pushing her wheelchair through the airport, tears escaped my eyes. It was a miracle to be traveling. Her dream had become a reality.

Though the travel physically knocked her down, precious time was spent sitting on the patio watching the shoreline. Lying by the pool while the kids splashed and played brought a smile to her face. Reclining in a lounge chair while her family snorkeled and paddle boarded brought a sense of unity and normalcy. Smelling the salty air and hearing the laughter of her loved ones offset the current trials, sprinkling them with delight.

One of Mom's specific requests for the trip was that we have private lessons from a hula-dancing instructor. How could we say no to that? At the hotel, the instructor taught us how to make leis and perform the Hukilau. We all donned hula skirts — even the men! Mom beamed watching her family try something new and entirely out of their comfort zone. Mom struggled to her feet and, for several minutes, hula-danced through her pain.

Though outwardly she was wasting away, inwardly she was being renewed day by day[010]. Back at home in Oregon... never giving in, never giving up, she would call to say, "I'm not dead yet! Where are we going today?" Picking strawberries, tasting olive oil made fresh at the factory, and going for long drives were highlights of her days. Attending quilt camp, visiting friends, and playing tour guide provided strength for the next bad day to come. Laughing, smiling, and saying sorry when she needed to, showed us her inner courage and humility. These were her final activities—the choice she made on how to leave this world. Loving people and living life to the fullest... until the very end.

### QUESTIONS:

Do you have a bucket list item that you'd like to see checked off? If so, what would that dream trip or experience look like?

What is one thing that would help you to have strength for the next bad day ahead?

Living life to the fullest for you will look different than it did for my mom or for the person sitting next to you at the doctor's office. What is one thing that you can do, think, or say to someone that would make the most of the opportunity you have today?

_____

_____

_____

_____

**PRAYER:**

_Dear Jesus, in the midst of this most difficult season, it is hard to live life to the fullest. The worries, the uncertainty, the appointments, the sickness, and the unmet expectations can drive us to become downtrodden, negative, and isolated. Help us today to embrace the people and opportunities before us. Give us dreams, and the stamina and provision to follow through with them. Help us to make lasting memories with those around us, no matter what today brings. Help us to live this life well. Amen._

# Glorious Unfolding (Part 1)

*Today I am grateful for long walks on the Maui beach with Michael before anyone else rises. This man has been my rock these past couple of months.*

**APRIL 17, 2015**

Songs bring emotion. Washing over us in unexpected ways, music can get embedded in our soul, leaving us flooded with emotions of many different kinds. Lyrics can make us dance, make us reminisce, and often make us cry.

As I was driving to the hospital one day, a song came on the radio—one I'd never heard before. I listened to the words and tears flooded my eyes. This song perfectly summed up Mom's cancer trial. So, later, as the whole family curled up on the couch in Hawaii, I shared the song along with the printed lyrics. We listened and read and agreed there was so much truth that compared to Mom's journey; "Glorious Unfolding" by Steven Curtis Chapman quickly became her theme song. It felt like it was written just for her.

## ASSIGNMENT & REFLECTION:

Instead of a longer journal entry today, I wanted to give you an assignment, not as a burden or another item on your to-do list, but as a way to create space for your heart to be encouraged. Head on over to the Resources page on our website (www.ourterminal.com/resources) and check out our Spotify playlist. Here you will find "Glorious Unfolding" along with a compilation of other songs that brought hope, peace, and comfort during my mom's terminal illness. I would love for these songs to remind you of truth as they did for me. If you have another song that feeds your soul, take time to listen to it today. Jot down some lines that resonate with your story, and record your thoughts below.

_____
_____
_____
_____
_____
_____
_____
_____
_____
_____
_____
_____
_____
_____
_____
_____
_____
_____

**PRAYER:**

*Father, you are a creative God. You give us the good gift of music. Music for times of joy and in times of lamenting. Thank you for this beautiful gift. Thank you for the ways that you remind us that you are still present in our story and for the hope that we can find in you. In our moments of doubt, help us to remember that you are working and that you use all things for good even if we don't understand. Help us to feel the emotions that creep up on us, even if they are big and overwhelming. Thank you for never leaving us. Amen.*

*Songs bring emotion.
Washing over us in unexpected
ways, music can get embedded in
our soul, leaving us flooded with
emotions of many different kinds.
Lyrics can make us dance,
make us reminisce, and
often make us cry.*

# Glorious Unfolding (Part 2)

Sometimes life just doesn't turn out like we want it to. Pain, illness, losses of all kinds, and death derail our future hopes. When unexpected circumstances arise, we wrestle over prayers we believe went unheard or plans that are now derailed. Sitting, spinning, over-analyzing, cycles of panic and worry rattle our thoughts. Questions like "How could God let this happen?" and "Why would God choose to cut someone's life short?" penetrate the deepest corners of our hearts.

At the core of the "Glorious Unfolding" song is the undeniable truth that God has greater plans for our story than we can see with our own eyes, beyond anything we can ever imagine. He looks through the lens of the fullness of time—eternity—while we can only see the small window of time in which we live. While God is omniscient (all-knowing) [011], omnipresent (present everywhere)[012], and eternal (existing before creation and for all time)[013], our knowledge and understanding are finite.

When it seems like God wrecks our perfect plans, allowing death and brokenness to come like a thief in the night, He still has glorious plans. Plans that were laid out well before our bodies ever entered the world[014]. Plans that just haven't yet been revealed.

A "Glorious Unfolding".

Long hours have been spent pondering what this means in Mom's life. Two months into her terminal disease, we understand that, barring a miracle, this disease will kill her. Having no clue how much time is left, or what her future holds, we are trying to wait with hopeful anticipation to see what God has in store. This song talks about how we simply need to hold onto the promises of God, the covenants He has made with us. Scripture is filled with truths like:

*"Come to me, all you who are weary and burdened, and I will give you rest."*

**MATTHEW 11:28–29**

*"He gives strength to the weary and increases the power of the weak. Even youths grow tired and weary, and young men stumble and fall; but those who hope in the Lord will renew their strength. They will soar on wings like eagles; they will run and not grow weary, they will walk and not be faint."*

**ISAIAH 40:29–40**

*"Peace I leave with you my peace I give you. I do not give to you as the world gives. Do not let your hearts be troubled and do not be afraid."*

**JOHN 14:27**

*"No, in all these things we are more than conquerors through him who loved us. For I am convinced that neither death nor life, neither angels nor demons, neither the present nor the future, nor any powers, neither height nor depth, nor anything else in all creative, will be able to separate us from the love of God that is in Christ Jesus or Lord."*

**ROMANS 8:37–39**

These are just a few of the promises God has given us. The Bible, the Word of God on paper, is filled with hundreds more. These promises are our constant; they are the stable, unbreakable foundation beneath the shaky ground under our feet.

God's plan over the course of history is that His people show the world His glory, grace, and love. His glory was on display when He rescued His people from a destitute future. Against all forces of nature, He parted the Red Sea, allowing the Israelites to escape from slavery in Egypt, eventually delivering them into the Promised Land[015]. His grace was on display through saving His chosen people from the hand of the bloodthirsty giant, Goliath[016]. God's love was displayed through our Savior's virgin birth[017], the miracles He performed[018], and ultimately His death and resurrection[019].

Though the pages of Scripture are complete, God is still writing His story of glory, grace, and love in the lives of each one of us. Through Mom's illness, her example of complete and wholehearted trust in God has encouraged others to have that same faith as their own. As people have rallied together, united by their love for her, the church has been displayed in beauty and true fellowship. Fear of death has been extinguished in the hearts of many because of Mom's peace. Eternity has been changed because of Mom's illness. Not just for her, but for many we will never know by name.

Mom's walk towards death, though tortuous to witness, is a reminder that God created us for citizenship in heaven, not on this earth. We are assigned a predetermined number of days. Our life is like a vapor[020] — here today and gone tomorrow. Heaven is eternal and forever, strolling in the presence of our God and Savior, there is no end to our life — perfected — there. No more tears. No more pain. No more sorrow[021]. THAT is what we were created to enjoy. This world is just a temporary stop, where we get to reflect His love to other people, drawing them closer to Him while living out the precious time we are given.

God is already touching so many people's lives through Mom's journey; we wait in humble expectation for His glorious unfolding yet to be revealed.

## QUESTIONS:

Do you have a song that has taken on special meaning during this terminal diagnosis? What do you love about it?

Ta lines

During a grief-filled, uncertain time like this, it can be really hard to see God's blessing in any part of it. Do you feel like you have been able to see His goodness in any big or small way? If so, list a few ways.

Do you feel like you can put your trust in an eternal life following death? Has this been something you have ever pondered before? If not, I encourage you to read the Invitation at the back of this journal or reach out to a hospital chaplain to speak with someone in person.

## PRAYER:

*Dear Heavenly Father, it is so hard to see your goodness when facing such a heartbreaking trial like this. There are days that we doubt your plan, and we wonder if there is any good that can come from this terminal illness. Help us to have an eternal perspective; to see things through your lens instead of our own. Help us to see you in the big and small blessings of today, and help us to trust you with our life after this illness. Show us your glory, Lord! Amen.*

# Being My Arms

*Today I am grateful for all the friends and family that are coming to visit Mom. It gives her joy and lifts her spirits to fellowship with her favorite people.*

MAY 7, 2015

In Exodus 17, Moses recounts the history of when the Amalekites went to battle against the Israelites. As Joshua went into the physical battle, Moses took Aaron and Hur to stand on top of a hill, the fight playing out in the valley below. Moses noticed that when his arms were strong and his staff was lifted high above his head, the Israelite Army would rally and victory seemed near.  But when the staff would lower, the army would appear defeated. As the battle wore on, Moses became tired, his arms slipping under the fatigue. Aaron and Hur, Moses' friends, sat Moses down upon a stone so he could rest, each picking up one end of the staff to hold it up for him. Moses was still holding on to this staff that contained the Lord's power... the same staff that struck a rock and produced flowing water and the same staff he held up to part the Red Sea to save his people and drown his enemies... but the physical ability to hold up the staff was coming from his friends. Did it have the same effect on the Israelite Army? Did they rally? You bet they did.

In Mom's life, we want this battle to press on because that means Mom is managing the cancer. We want to fight and engage the struggle. Relative health and "good days" are the goal, but with it comes a prolonged, never-ending hardship. Tired and weary, weak and struggling, we cannot do this journey alone.

Moses had Aaron and Hur. My family has all our dear friends, extended family, neighbors, church class, and hospital staff. They have held our arms up while the battle has raged on for over three months... carpooling my children, cleaning Mom's house, and paying to have someone clean mine. Sending cards, flowers, prayer blankets, and food, their love has nurtured and built our stamina. These people have sat by my mom's bedside so I could have a night at home and have prayed over her as if she were their own mother. Flying thousands of miles to spend days with her, they have shared old memories while making new ones in the process. Despite any personal uncomfort, these souls let me cry and let Mom talk about her memorial service. They sent me texts reminding me of God's faithfulness while simultaneously lamenting the tragedy of battle-weary days. Some embraced a woman they hardly know into their lives as they helped her make quilts as keepsakes for my girls. Most of all, these beautiful people have prayed. Prayed for good days, for little pain, for peace beyond understanding, and for endurance. They have prayed for sweet family time, for important conversations, and for grace. They prayed us to Hawaii and back, and for God's glory to shine when human understanding dictates otherwise.

*Without these amazing people, this battle would be too much. Without God this fight would be impossible.*

Without these amazing people, this battle would be too much. Without God this fight would be impossible. Our gratitude for the meals, childcare, encouragement, and prayer; our thankfulness for their courage and strength is impossible to overstate. While the war battles on, we are grateful beyond words to have these people on our side.

Our people are our arms. Because of them we can press on.

### QUESTIONS:

Do you have an Aaron and Hur in your life, someone who is walking close beside you? Who are they and how has their presence or help made such an impact on your life?

_____

_____

_____

_____

If you don't have people who you can count on during this time, is there anyone that you can reach out to ask for some help? A local church, a neighbor, a coworker, or extended family might be a great place to start. Jot down some ideas here.

What part of this diagnosis has been the hardest for you? Is it the physical toll it takes, the emotions that come with it, or the spiritual wrestling? Is there someone you could share these thoughts with?

What is one thing that someone could do for you today that would make today feel a little bit lighter? Who is a person you could ask to help you with this?

**PRAYER:**

*Oh Jesus, we can't fight the battle alone. We desperately need a community of people to hold up our arms when we cannot find the strength. Would you please bring people into our lives to help carry the heavy load and would you show us who can walk this road alongside us. Thank you, God, for the people already standing with us and for the way that you are our ultimate strength and shield. Amen.*

# Beauty from a Hospital Bed

*Today I am grateful for hospitals and pain medicines.*

**MAY 28, 2015**

Today I walked through the hospital corridors for what felt like the 1,000th time in four months. Sometimes, Mom seems to take two steps forward and one giant leap back, all in the matter of a few days.

Yesterday I awoke in the middle of the night to my phone ringing; Mom was in so much pain and throwing up violently. The only option was to get her to the hospital as quickly as possible. She was at the lowest point we've seen her since the original diagnosis and needed to be admitted to the oncology floor once again. After getting some medication and subsequent rest, today dawned a bit brighter. As Mom lay in her hospital bed this afternoon, a hospital staff member walked in to take over the shift. Instantly recognizing her from a previous hospital visit, Mom began getting reacquainted by saying, "I hope this doesn't come across as rude, but weren't you pregnant last time I saw you?" The women's smile faltered as she explained that her baby had been lost to miscarriage. Tears welled up in my eyes as I watched Mom pour grace and blessing upon her, giving hope for tomorrow in the midst of her pain. Entering into understanding as a fellow mom who had lost babies in her early years, Mom reached out across a line that can feel silent and alone. As a silent bystander to this special encounter, I sat amazed at the care and tenderness Mom displayed. It was beautiful.

This moment sums up who Mom is at her best. Though experiencing devastating circumstances of her own, she could still comfort another woman, fifty years younger, in a pain that is just as real to her as my mom's illness is to us. It was almost as if God knew that young woman needed Mom to be in that bed for this special reason, just for today.

## QUESTIONS:

Are there any details about the care facility or the staff that stand out to you; observations or names you want to remember in the future?

_____

_____

_____

_____

Have you met anyone lately whose story you can relate to? If so, how were you able to encourage one another?

_____

_____

_____

_____

Is there a pain in your past that you have seen God use to comfort someone going through a similar loss? If so, describe who it was and how you were able to help.

_____

_____

_____

_____

## PRAYER:

_Dear Lord, thank you for the way you can continue to use us to reach other people in their time of need. Thank you for your promise that our current trials will be redeemed and that you will work out all things for good in your time. Would you bring us someone today who needs our smile, or kind words, or our presence. Give us the ability to be a joy and a light to those around us, even in our deepest pain. Thank you for the ways you still show us that our days matter and that our lives have purpose for your Kingdom. Amen._

*"Tears welled up in my eyes as I watched Mom pour grace and blessing upon her, giving hope for tomorrow in the midst of her pain.*

# Beautifully Broken

*Today I am grateful that Mom hasn't lost her trademark snow-white hair, despite all the chemo pumped into her body.*

**MAY 31, 2015**

Thirty-four years of marriage down the drain. Receiving that call one morning while cradling my infant daughter felt like a slap across the face. Processing Mom's cries of immense sorrow, I could almost hear her tears spilling over the receiver. All these years. All these memories. All this love. Gone.

Sometimes people make mistakes. Choices are made that cost a lot. Mess-ups can't always be undone with a simple "I'm sorry." The first couple of years following my parent's sudden separation and eventual divorce were ugly. Mom was enraged, to the point of almost losing her sanity some days. Hearing details I never wanted to hear, my heart ached for the loss of our family. Worry and confusion of what Mom's future now held kept my husband and me up at night. Fervently praying that God would somehow work through this brokenness and bring healing, we never could have imagined the full extent He would answer that prayer.

Slowly, over time, my parents began to communicate again. The birth of a new daughter for me, and a cross-country move for my sister forced them to continue to be a team. Further down the road, health challenges deepened their dependence on one another. With their children living out of state, they leaned on each other when cataracts needed fixing or small procedures arose. When Dad was diagnosed with prostate cancer a few years ago, Mom opened her home to him, helping with post-op protocol and feeding him so he could regain his strength. Neighbors began to ask questions like, "How could she pour out love on him after the grueling divorce they had?" or "Why would she call to check on him?" or "Why would she ask him for help when she needed it?" Their post-divorce relationship was perplexing, complicated, and inexplicable to everyone but themselves. It was beautiful.

One evening, Mom and Dad sat across the dinner table from one another at her neighborhood clubhouse. With tears in her eyes she told Dad she forgave him. For everything. Telling him that she valued their friendship, she was grateful they had been able to move forward and thankful he had contributed to keeping the family unit together and whole. Dad now says that this moment was a pivotal juncture in his own faith. Mom extended forgiveness to him, just as Christ does every day for us[022].

*God redeemed their relationship in a powerful and redemptive way that was a testimony to those around them.*

When Mom made both her temporary and permanent moves to Oregon, Dad was the first to offer to drive her cross-country. With four full days alone in the car together, they cherished that time. Good conversation materialized, nice visits to family took place along the trip, and healing continued to transpire. After Mom's terminal diagnosis, Dad traveled from Texas to Oregon almost every month to stay with her; the visits were treasures to Mom, and also allowed me to have some reprieve. Dad knew Mom in a way the rest of us didn't. For so many years they had been life partners, knowing the intimate details of each other's personalities and preferences. Dad could provide her comfort and peace in these final months in a way no one else could.

In some ways, I think their relationship at the end of Mom's life was healthier than when they were married. Both were coming into their own faith, able to see life through a clearer lens, knowing themselves and one another in a fresh and more genuine way. My wish was that they could have come to these revelations while their marriage still hung in the balance, but that wasn't their story. God redeemed their relationship in a powerful and redemptive way that was a testimony to those around them.

Beautifully broken is the phrase I use to describe Mom and Dad's relationship—broken in the sense that their marriage failed, ending in a tragic way. The wake of suffering impacted the entire family, and devastation and stress followed for years. But beautiful because the ending was simply that. Extending and receiving forgiveness and having genuine concern for one another, Mom and Dad were willing to chart a new future during the time they had left together.

I will be forever grateful that my parents chose to reconcile early so Mom's last months could be filled with beauty, companionship, and love. When death is forthcoming and time is running out, forgiveness can still be given or received regardless of the length of time passed or the depth of the wound.

## QUESTIONS:

Why is forgiveness so hard? What gets in the way of helping us to forgive another person?

Is there anyone in your life that you need to forgive? What steps can you take to extend forgiveness to that person?

Is there anyone that you need to ASK forgiveness from, anyone you have hurt in the past and need to apologize to? I encourage you to take your first step in seeking reconciliation.

## PRAYER:

*Oh God, forgiveness is so hard. Our wounds from past hurts run deep, and sometimes no amount of time can mend that brokenness. We know that, through you alone, we can extend true forgiveness despite all that has happened, just as you have forgiven us through Christ. Help me to extend forgiveness today to anyone in my life who needs to hear those words from me. Help me to offer grace and to be bold enough to say it aloud. Please bring to mind anyone whom I have hurt, who needs my apology, and may they have a softened heart to forgive me in return. Thank you for being our example of true forgiveness. Help us to follow your lead. Amen.*

# Choose Your Own Adventure

*Today I am grateful Michael takes Mom to the ER in the middle of the night so I can get some rest.*

**JUNE 3, 2015**

When I was a kid, it was a great day in the school library when they had a new *Choose Your Own Adventure* book on the shelf. These books appealed to me because if I didn't like how the first ending came to pass, a different way was available to explore. I could *choose* my own ending. What a great concept! I used to stress about which path to take initially, even though a "redo" remained if necessary. After all, it wasn't real life, was it? And so I could start over...

There have been many times in my life I wish I could have a "choose-my-own-adventure" ending. Things have happened, or choices have been made, resulting in consequences or outcomes I wouldn't have picked. If only I could scroll back fifty pages and try a different way, perhaps the ending would be less shocking or less painful.

Where is the redo option in Mom's current cancer twist?

Mom's new adventure to Oregon started out happy. Her previous cancer had gone into remission and she was no longer sick. All was well. Feeling like a new chapter had opened, she embraced the change with enthusiasm. The adventure she signed up for included lots of babysitting dates, volunteering at school, planting a vegetable garden, and playtime in the incredible surrounding nature this fresh locale had to offer.

Three months into this new routine, our family turned the page to a chapter we couldn't have expected. Mom's terminal cancer diagnosis brought great amounts of pain, staining the pages of an adventure that was supposed to be happy. We didn't

> *The only decision we got to make was that we would continue to turn the pages, one by one, entrusting that the ending would be redeemed, believing that her story was not yet over.*

get to choose the next events and we couldn't predict the upcoming twists and turns. We weren't going to get a "redo." The only decision we got to make was that we would continue to turn the pages, one by one, entrusting that the ending would be redeemed, believing that her story was not yet over.

Mom's new adventure moving here was supposed to look different. What we dreamed it would be looks nothing like the reality of what it is. But if I had the choice to rewrite the narrative, erasing the story of the past few months, I don't think I would. I *have learned* so much about what it means to love another person. I *have learned* what selfless living really feels like. I *have learned* how we can glorify God in our pain in ways we can't when life is good. I *have learned* to keep my treasures in jars of clay[023], hoping for what is unseen more than what is seen. I *have learned* that sometimes the adventures we want the least might be the ones that are ironically best for our own faith journey and that of those around us. I *have learned* true joy in the midst of great pain. I *have learned* to let my guard down and show others my emotions. I *have learned* to receive help. I *have learned* that every day is truly a gift. I *have learned* to be content... no matter what[024].

I hope that the next time a new adventure arises, I won't be so afraid to take the plunge and turn the next page. This adventure of Mom's has shown me to never be afraid of a plot twist. Because, sometimes, even the painful ones are full of joyous surprises.

## QUESTIONS:

What did life look like pre-diagnosis for you or your loved one? This can include hobbies, classes, appointments, standing family or friend gatherings, annual trips, etc.

Can you see any unexpected blessings or gifts that have come despite your current circumstance? List a few below.

_____

_____

_____

_____

Looking back at your life, are there any parts you wish you could go back and rewrite? (For example: handling a situation differently, taking a risk you chose not to, not taking a risk you did choose to, reconciling with a person, etc.)

_____

_____

_____

_____

**PRAYER:**

*Dear Jesus, it is hard to accept that we can't control the end of this road we are traveling. We confess that we struggle with your plan and that we yearn for a different ending. Please help us today to be able to loosen our grip and to hand this journey back over to you. It's so hard to not be able to change our current suffering. Help us, Lord Jesus, to trust you as the Author and Perfecter of our lives. Help us to see your goodness in a story we hoped you'd never write. Amen.*

# Hope Deferred

*Today I am grateful for the harpist that came by the hospital room to play "I'll Fly Away," "It Is Well with My Soul," and "Amazing Grace" over Mom. It drew the first smile we have seen from her in days.*

**JULY 12, 2015**

Hope can be a tricky thing. Hope can make us feel alive, quickening our pulse, spurring us to go out and change the world. In contrast, hope can feel like grasping for straws when the future seems scary and uncertain—the only word we can use when conventional logic fails us.

For me, only my faith in Jesus gives me the ability to have hope in the midst of this impossible trial. Even if it feels like the whole world is crashing down around me, faith in my good God can buoy me amidst the chaos. Hebrews 11:1 says, "For faith is being sure of what we hope for and certain of what we do not see. This is what the ancients were commended for." The chapter continues to describe people who did not receive the things promised, only welcoming them from a distance. For example, Abraham trusted God with the life of his only son. Jacob blessed his sons as he leaned on his staff dying. Moses' parents hid him for three months because they knew he was set apart for God's purposes. Rahab risked her life to help the spies, thus saving her life and the lives of those she loved. Person after person is listed for their faith, even when they didn't get to receive the intended blessing or see the fulfillment of their dreams.

Mom's faith statement could read... "By faith, Nancy, who faced certain death, lived large, loved deeply, and held onto God's promises with unwavering conviction. Never taking her eyes off heaven, she continued to live out the purposes God set in advance for her to do."

Hebrews 11:39 says, "They were all commended for their faith, yet none of them received what they had promised. God has planned something better for us, so that only together with us would they be made perfect." Mom isn't getting the full ninety plus years she had wanted. She isn't getting to see

*But God, in His great mercy, has something much sweeter in store for her.*

her children age into late adulthood, or her grandchildren grow up. She isn't getting to come to Oregon and "play" like she had planned. But God, in His great mercy, has something much sweeter in store for her. She is about to receive a kingdom that can never be shaken, where sorrow and pain are forgotten, and where a new body and an eternal home await her arrival. She is in the final stages of trading in her earthly tent for her heavenly dwelling[025]. Ready and willing to give her spirit to her heavenly Father, we trust He is near; and we learn from her "Hall of Faith" devotion to the very end.

## QUESTIONS:

Is there someone in your life that you would consider a "Hall of Faith" person? What makes (or made) their faith stand out to you as extra special?

How have you seen God grow your faith through your life and circumstances?

If you could write your own faith summary, what would it say?

**PRAYER:**

*God, we thank you for the faithful people that have walked this earth before us, especially those who have impacted our lives in a personal way. We declare today that we want to be listed among those men and women who have trusted in God despite their unmet hopes or dreams gone astray. We want others to be able to witness our trust in you despite our current suffering. Help us to be people of deep faith, trust, hope, and perseverance. Help us to run this race you have set before us with grace, honesty, and an eternal perspective. We trust you, Lord. Amen.*

# Do Not Delay

*Today I am thankful that our hope is in heaven.*

**JULY 20, 2015**

My warrior mama. So brave. So strong. So faithful. Never dreaming she would still be on this earth, her fight continues to the very end. Today I am praying that God would reveal to me whatever I need to learn from this time of waiting. I fully trust that He has good plans for this interim. Because why else would He be asking Mom to wait for heaven?

> *Because why else would He be asking Mom to wait for heaven?*

These three words, Do Not Delay, are scribbled over and over again in my journal symbolizing the toughest trial of our life. Today my prayer has been for God to not delay in taking Mom to heaven. Though I will never be ready for Mom to leave my presence on this earth, the pain and agony of watching her hang in the balance of life and death is excruciating. Several days ago, Mom told the pastor from our church that she was unafraid and ready to go, soundly muting the argument that the physical fight is still in her.

Sitting by her side day in and day out, I trust God has a good purpose in this time of waiting; but it's hard for me not to wonder why He has delayed. One deeply felt purpose is that my sister, Emily, got to faithfully sit beside Mom through the day and sleep in the recliner through the night. Through these long, arduous hours, she is now able to fully release Mom to heaven. For my own heart, I have come to fully accept Mom's departure from my side, yearning for her to stay, yet trusting that this is God's plan and that it will be okay. It is hard to let go, terrifying and hurt-filled, but I am ready for Mom's heavy burden to end.

Exactly a week ago Mom was put on hospice and fluid and nourishment were slowed down as her body couldn't process them any longer. Mom has always been a fighter, and though her body is shutting down, her spirit is still pressing on. Over the past week her family has gotten to experience some closure. Watching her release control, prepared to say goodbye to this world, our hearts have embraced her wishes. It's hard. It stings. It's soul-wrenching. But, it is her time.

So, my heart cries out to you, dear Jesus. Extend your hand to her today; let her leave the pain, sorrow, tears, and suffering of this world. Welcome her into your pearly gates, complete with a refashioned, eternal body. Allow her to sit in Your presence as she desires to be.

*"Then your light will break forth like the dawn, and your healing will quickly appear, then your righteousness will go before you and the glory of the Lord will be your rear guard."*

**ISAIAH 58:8**

DO NOT DELAY.

### QUESTIONS:

How is the waiting and wondering wearing on your own heart?

Do you feel restless over what is to come or do you have peace in the unknown?

Do you believe in an eternal place? If so, what do you think it will be like? How do you get there?

_____

_____

_____

_____

**PRAYER:**

_Oh, dear Jesus. We yearn for your closeness today. Though none of us know when our last day on this earth will be, we sense that you are close at hand. We ask that you help us to release control and allow you to usher in your presence in a near and deep way. And while we may feel restless about what is to come, may you show us your goodness in each of our days. Amen._

# Leaving The Terminal

*Today I am grateful that, though my heart is fragile, it is full of hope. I see more than ever that death was never part of God's original design. I am thankful we can be restored even though death still comes.*

Several hours after writing the last journal entry, "Do Not Delay", my mom left me, us, this world. I was by her side. Michael was by mine. It was shortly after that Snickers bar. I'm glad I saw it and thought to purchase it from the vending machine, sharing one more memory of old, while turning it into a new one. We celebrated one last moment of "us being us"… and then she took her first breath in her eternal home.

After spending a few minutes by her side, I summoned her favorite nurse, Arley, who, by God's grace, was working late that night. I shared the news that Mom had died. As we walked back to the room, she encouraged me to take as much time as I needed by Mom's side. Strange as it might seem, I felt released to start packing up our personal items and then head home. My bedside vigil over the past twelve days felt complete. Mom, as I knew her, wasn't there any longer. As Michael and I walked out of the room for the very last time, I looked back over my shoulder. Tears slipped from my eyes as I whispered one final "goodbye".

\*\*\*

Thank you, Mom, for everything. Your sacrificial love, contagious fun, and deep conviction have molded me into the woman I am today.  The earth is changed because of your courage to walk this journey to heaven. Your legacy will reach people and places yet to be seen. I can't wait for the day I get to see you again.

# REFLECTION

# Invitation

# Invitation

Dear Friend,

As you have traveled through the pages of this journal, my biggest prayer is that you have encountered the idea of HOPE in every nook and cranny of our story. I want to tell you why my mom and I both were able to have hope even though Mom's time on earth was ending and there was nothing we could do about it. Mom was a Christian, I am a Christian, and we didn't believe that life ends after death on earth. Here's why...

## GOD CREATED ALL THINGS

God created the earth and everything in it. This includes you and me. God created us in His image (Genesis 1:26) and with a purpose and a mission (Genesis 2:15). He also created us for relationship, with each other and with Him (Genesis 3:8). When He looked at all He made, He said that it was GOOD.

## THE PROBLEM

God created us to be in relationship with Him, but there was a problem. The first people God made, Adam and Eve, disobeyed God's one and only rule for them. They ate fruit from the tree of the knowledge of good and evil because they wanted to be more like God. Their pride and greed led to disobedience and *sin* entered the world. Sin separates us from God because God is *holy*... He is perfect. He can't be in a relationship with people who are not because it would tarnish his holiness.

When Adam and Eve sinned, everything changed. One of the most profound and painful things that entered our world was death. "When Adam sinned, sin entered the world. Adam's sin brought death, so death spread to everyone, for everyone sinned." (Romans 5:12) *Death was not in God's original plan.*

And just as Adam and Eve's sin messed everything up, our sin has the same consequence. Whether it's lying, stealing, jealousy, lust, selfish ambition, or gossip, we all fall short of the glory of a holy God (Romans 3:23). We all go the wrong way, and nothing we do in life can bridge the divide between us and our perfect Creator.

## THE SOLUTION

I am happy to tell you... there IS an answer. This problem has already been solved! While we cannot ever be "good enough" to have a relationship with God on our own, God loves us so much that *He provided a solution for us.*

God put a great plan into motion. Here entered the bridge for our great divide. Here entered a sacrifice for all the sins we have ever committed and the ones to come. Jesus Christ, God's only Son, came to earth as a baby. This is why Christians celebrate Christmas... the birth of Jesus. He was fully God AND fully man, experiencing the same temptations and struggles we face today; yet He lived a perfect, sinless life on this earth, something no one else could ever do.

After He spent 33 years on earth and taught thousands upon thousands about the one true God, some religious and political rulers of the day became afraid. Jesus was sound in his beliefs. He spoke purely and convincingly. He threatened their control. During Jesus' ministry on earth, he taught crowds of people about God, performed miracles in front of many, and loved the outcast and the broken. He spoke purely and convincingly about the Kingdom of God, becoming a threat to the religious and political leaders of the time. In the end, Jesus was falsely accused, ridiculed, beaten, and ultimately died a brutal death. But because he was also God, that wasn't the end of the story...


## VICTORY

If the story ended with death, you could just put Jesus into a category with a handful of people who have claimed to be the savior of the world only to die and prove that they are not. Jesus did die, the difference is that He didn't stay dead! Three days after being buried in a sealed and guarded tomb, the grave was found to be empty. Jesus had risen from the dead! He was fully alive and completely healed. Over the next few weeks, hundreds of people who had seen Him die, saw Him living again. Sin and death were defeated at last!

And so, Jesus, who was fully God AND fully man served as a perfect sacrifice. While innocent, He died in our place. Instead of us paying a penalty for all the wrongs we commit against a perfect God, Jesus did it for us. Once and for all, there was declared victory over death. Once and for all, there was a way we could have a relationship in this life with our perfect Creator even though we ourselves are not perfect.

And now, Jesus is reunited with God in a place called heaven.

When we die on this earth, we can spend eternity in heaven with God because of Christ's sacrifice on the cross for our sins. All we have to do is believe in Jesus Christ as our Savior. *THIS is the hope I have been talking about.*


## IT IS NEVER TOO LATE


You might be reading this today and realizing that your time on this earth is short. Be encouraged, my friend. If you still have breath in your lungs, you can still believe in Jesus Christ. What that means for you is that when you take your final breath, whether it is next year or tomorrow morning, you will immediately be ushered into the presence of your loving God for eternity. Putting your faith in Jesus means that heaven is waiting for you when your life comes to an end.

Heaven is an amazing and beautiful place where we will experience the fullness of God, and a place where we will enjoy rest, peace, and joy that only He offers. All the pain you have experienced will be replaced with peace. All the death and darkness will be replaced with life and light. All our loss and sorrow will be replaced with complete fulfillment and joy.

Revelation 21:4 promises,

*"He will wipe every tear from their eyes. There will be no more death or mourning or crying or pain, for the old order of things has passed away."*

You don't have to have all your faith questions answered before you place your faith in Jesus, you just have to SURRENDER your control. To say that you cannot ever be perfect and that you believe Jesus paid that debt for you. Jesus is waiting for you to say "yes" to Him.

If you are caring for someone you love, and this road has felt impossible, know that Jesus is waiting to help carry your burden for you. Matthew 11:28-30 says,

> *"Come to me, all you who are weary and burdened, and I will give you rest. Take my yoke upon you and learn from me, for I am gentle and humble in heart, and you will find rest for your souls. For my yoke is easy and my burden is light."*

You don't have to walk this alone. By placing your faith in Jesus, you will be given the power of the Holy Spirit... this is the third part in the "Trinity" you might have heard of. God, Jesus, and the Holy Spirit are one, yet with different roles. The Holy Spirit is a helper and a friend who will guide you in decisions and comfort you in grief. You will have access to the joy of the Lord and it can be your supernatural strength. Your road of grief ahead is heavy; but, with Jesus, beauty and purpose can be a part of it.

Bottom line, God wants a relationship with you. He wants to give you rest, peace, strength. He wants to give you Himself.

## TODAY CAN BE THE DAY

If you are ready to make that decision, would you pray with me...

*"Dear God, I know that you created me and that you love me. I understand that I am not perfect or can ever be "good enough" to have a relationship with you on my own. Forgive me of the things I have done in my life that haven't pleased you, things I have said or done that have hurt those around me. I believe that Jesus took the punishment I deserve for my sin and died as a perfect sacrifice for me. I believe that you, Jesus, didn't stay dead. I believe that You were raised to life again and that you proclaimed victory over death once and for all. I want to start my life with Jesus today. I believe! In the strong name of Jesus, Amen."*

If you prayed this prayer today, please share this good news with someone you love. If you feel like you don't have anyone to tell, please tell us at Our Terminal. We would love to celebrate with you! **You can reach us at contact@ourterminal.com.**

Do you already know Christ as your personal Savior? If you do, then we celebrate that with you. I encourage you to write down how you came to know the Lord or to share it with a loved one. Include ways you have seen God show Himself faithful and the ways you have experienced Him through the seasons of your life. Your faith story will bless generations to come.

# In Memoriam:

This journal was funded, in part, by generous donors who gave in memory or in honor of their loved ones. We are so grateful for their support and feel privileged to include these names within the pages of this book.

**Col. David Braden**

**Dr. James Braden**

**Becky Cranmer**

**Rose Ann Fischer Ilse**

**Cate George**

**Ret. Col. Earl Hoag**

**Sharon Hossack**

**Sandy Jeffcoat**

**Nancy Lanford**

**Cory Looper**

**Kathy Lovely**

**Lucy Lozier & all Hope Babies**

**Barbara Pogue**

**Anita L. Ray**

**Opal Reddin**

**Sherry Rouse**

**Barbara Shaw**

# Journeying Through Terminal Illness With Hope & Each Other

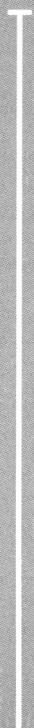

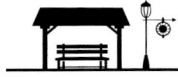

# OUR TERMINAL

Our Terminal began in 2018 as a nonprofit devoted to offering resources and hope for individuals and families facing terminal illness. We do this by providing truth-filled devotionals and online resources and also through community partnerships. Through these materials and connections, Our Terminal desires to offer support to others — like you — walking the same path we've walked. We want you to know that there can be hope in the middle of this unimaginable time. We believe that each person's story matters and that no one should walk through a terminal diagnosis alone.

If you have found comfort, hope, or encouragement through any of our resources, whether online or in print, please consider making a donation* to Our Terminal? Your generous support will help more families like yours have access to God's truth during this last chapter of life.

**To learn more about Our Terminal and the resources we offer,**

**visit us at: ourterminal.com**

[01]James 1:22 Do not merely listen to the word, and so deceive yourselves. Do what it says.

[02]John 15:13 Greater love has no one than this: to lay down one's life for one's friends.

[03]Matthew 7:12 So in everything, do to others what you would have them do to you, for this sums up the Law and the Prophets.

[04]Mark 12:29-31 "The most important one," answered Jesus, "is this: 'Hear, O Israel: The Lord our God, the Lord is one. Love the Lord your God with all your heart and with all your soul and with all your mind and with all your strength.' The second is this: 'Love your neighbor as yourself.' There is no commandment greater than these."

[05]Romans 8:31-39 What, then, shall we say in response to these things? If God is for us, who can be against us? He who did not spare his own Son, but gave him up for us all—how will he not also, along with him, graciously give us all things? Who will bring any charge against those whom God has chosen? It is God who justifies. Who then is the one who condemns? No one. Christ Jesus who died—more than that, who was raised to life—is at the right hand of God and is also interceding for us. Who shall separate us from the love of Christ? Shall trouble or hardship or persecution or famine or nakedness or danger or sword? As it is written:
    "For your sake we face death all day long;
    we are considered as sheep to be slaughtered."
    No, in all these things we are more than conquerors through him who loved us. For I am convinced that neither death nor life, neither angels nor demons, neither the present nor the future, nor any powers, neither height nor depth, nor anything else in all creation, will be able to separate us from the love of God that is in Christ Jesus our Lord.

[06]Isaiah 40:12 Who has measured the waters in the hollow of his hand,
    or with the breadth of his hand marked off the heavens?
    Who has held the dust of the earth in a basket,
    or weighed the mountains on the scales
    and the hills in a balance?

[07]Hebrews 13:5 Keep your lives free from the love of money and be content with what you have, because God has said, "Never will I leave you; never will I forsake you."

[08]Jeremiah 29:11 "For I know the plans I have for you," declares the Lord, "plans to prosper you and not to harm you, plans to give you hope and a future."

[09]Genesis 16:13 She gave this name to the Lord who spoke to her: "You are the God who sees me," for she said, "I have now seen the One who sees me."

[010]2 Corinthians 4:16 Therefore we do not lose heart. Though outwardly we are wasting away, yet inwardly we are being renewed day by day.

[011]Psalm 147:5 Great is our Lord and mighty in power; his understanding has no limit.

[012]Psalm 139:7-10 Where can I go from your Spirit?
   Where can I flee from your presence?
   If I go up to the heavens, you are there;
   if I make my bed in the depths, you are there.
   If I rise on the wings of the dawn,
   if I settle on the far side of the sea,
   even there your hand will guide me,
   your right hand will hold me fast.
   If I say, "Surely the darkness will hide me
   and the light become night around me,"
   even the darkness will not be dark to you;
   the night will shine like the day,
   for darkness is as light to you.

[013]Revelation 22:13 I am the Alpha and the Omega, the First and the Last, the Beginning and the End.

[014]Psalm 139:16 Your eyes saw my unformed body; all the days ordained for me were written in your book before one of them came to be.

[015]Exodus 14:21-22 Then Moses stretched out his hand over the sea, and all that night the Lord drove the sea back with a strong east wind and turned it into dry land. The waters were divided, and the Israelites went through the sea on dry ground, with a wall of water on their right and on their left.

[016]1 Samuel 17:45-47 David said to the Philistine, "You come against me with sword and spear and javelin, but I come against you in the name of the Lord Almighty, the God of the armies of Israel, whom you have defied. This day the Lord will deliver you into my hands, and I'll strike you down and cut off your head. This very day I will give the carcasses of the Philistine army to the birds and the wild animals, and the whole world will know that there is a God in Israel. All those gathered here will know that it is not by sword or spear that the Lord saves; for the battle is the Lord's, and he will give all of you into our hands."

[017]Isaiah 7:14 Therefore the Lord himself will give you a sign: The virgin will conceive and give birth to a son, and will call him Immanuel.

[018]Mark 5:25-34 And a woman was there who had been subject to bleeding for twelve years. She had suffered a great deal under the care of many doctors and had spent all she had, yet instead of getting better she grew worse. When she heard about Jesus, she came up behind him

in the crowd and touched his cloak, because she thought, "If I just touch his clothes, I will be healed." Immediately her bleeding stopped and she felt in her body that she was freed from her suffering.

At once Jesus realized that power had gone out from him. He turned around in the crowd and asked, "Who touched my clothes?"

"You see the people crowding against you," his disciples answered, "and yet you can ask, 'Who touched me?' "

But Jesus kept looking around to see who had done it. Then the woman, knowing what had happened to her, came and fell at his feet and, trembling with fear, told him the whole truth. He said to her, "Daughter, your faith has healed you. Go in peace and be freed from your suffering."

[019]Luke 24:6-7 He is not here; he has risen! Remember how he told you, while he was still with you in Galilee: "The Son of Man must be delivered over to the hands of sinners, be crucified and on the third day be raised again."

[020]James 4:14 Why, you do not even know what will happen tomorrow. What is your life? You are a mist that appears for a little while and then vanishes.

[021]Revelation 21:4 He will wipe every tear from their eyes. There will be no more death or mourning or crying or pain, for the old order of things has passed away.

[022]1 John 1:9 If we confess our sins, he is faithful and just and will forgive us our sins and purify us from all unrighteousness.

[023]2 Corinthians 4:7 But we have this treasure in jars of clay to show that this all-surpassing power is from God and not from us.

[024]Philippians 4:11 I am not saying this because I am in need, for I have learned to be content whatever the circumstances.

[025]2 Corinthians 5:1 For we know that if the earthly tent we live in is destroyed, we have a building from God, an eternal house in heaven, not built by human hands.

# REFLECTION & PRAYERS

## REFLECTION & PRAYERS

# REFLECTION & PRAYERS

# REFLECTION & PRAYERS

# REFLECTION & PRAYERS

# REFLECTION & PRAYERS

## REFLECTION & PRAYERS

# REFLECTION & PRAYERS

# REFLECTION & PRAYERS

# REFLECTION & PRAYERS